SAMANTHA PETEREIN

Rooted in Healing: An Introduction to Herbs and Rituals for Wellness

This book was professionally typeset on Reedsy.
Find out more at reedsy.com

Contents

Introduction

The Power of Herbs and Rituals in Healing

In a world that often feels chaotic and overwhelming, it can be easy to lose our connection to the things that keep us balanced—our bodies, our breath, the simple moments of stillness that bring us back to ourselves. The truth is, healing isn't something we have to search for far and wide. It's all around us, found in nature's quiet wisdom and in the simple, intentional acts of self-care that we can create every day.

This guide is a gentle reminder that healing is accessible to all of us. It's a way of coming home to ourselves, rooted in the timeless wisdom of herbs and the nurturing power of rituals. Whether you're just beginning your journey into holistic wellness or have been practicing for years, the herbs and self-care practices in this book offer simple, practical tools for grounding, revitalizing, and restoring balance to your life.

I created this guide not only from my own journey of healing but also from a deep desire to help others find their own paths to wellness. Over the years, I've learned that healing is rarely a straight line. It's a process of learning to listen to our bodies, trusting our intuition, and finding comfort in the small rituals that bring us back to center.

Healing Herbs and Rituals: A Natural Partnership

Throughout the pages of this book, you'll discover the power of healing herbs that have been used for centuries to calm the mind, soothe the body, and nourish the spirit. These herbs, paired with simple self-care rituals, create a powerful partnership that supports both physical and emotional wellness. Each herb brings its own unique properties, offering something different depending on what your body and mind need.

In this guide, you'll learn how to:

- Use herbs to ground yourself when life feels overwhelming.
- Incorporate energizing herbs to uplift and restore your vitality.
- Create rituals that help you find moments of peace and clarity in your day.
- Support emotional healing and stress relief through herbal remedies.
- Find simple, nurturing ways to care for your skin and body using nature's gifts.

Each section of this book is designed to give you practical, easy-to-follow steps for integrating herbal remedies and rituals into your daily life. These aren't complicated or time-consuming practices—they're small, intentional acts that can be woven into the rhythm of your day to bring a sense of balance, peace, and connection.

A Personal Journey to Healing

My own path to healing has been winding and filled with its share of challenges, but through it all, nature has been my greatest teacher. The herbs and rituals in this book have been a part of my personal healing journey, and now I offer them to you. Whether you're seeking emotional support, physical relief, or simply a deeper connection to yourself, I hope this guide serves as a gentle companion on your journey.

As you explore the pages ahead, remember that healing is not a destination. It's a practice—a way of being. With each herb you use, with each ritual you create, may you come closer to finding balance, peace, and wholeness.

Let's begin.

1

Grounding with Herbal Remedies

Grounding: Why It's Essential for Wellness

In today's fast-paced world, it's easy to feel unsteady—like we're constantly being pulled in multiple directions. Grounding brings us back to the present moment, helps us reconnect with ourselves, and gives us the stability we need to feel balanced, both mentally and physically. Just as roots keep a tree anchored to the earth, grounding practices and herbs help us anchor ourselves in our bodies and minds.

Whether you're feeling anxious, overwhelmed, or simply scattered, incorporating grounding rituals and herbs into your daily routine can make a profound difference in how you feel. The herbs highlighted in this section are known for their calming and stabilizing properties, helping you to reconnect with your body, reduce stress, and find peace in the present moment.

Herbs for Grounding: Calming the Mind and Body

Chamomile (Matricaria chamomilla)

- Properties: Chamomile is well-known for its soothing, calming effects. It helps ease tension, calm the nervous system, and reduce anxiety, making it a perfect herb for grounding rituals.
- How to Use: Brew chamomile as a simple tea to drink at the end of a long day, or add chamomile flowers to a warm bath for a calming, grounding experience.
- Practical Tip: Try sipping a cup of chamomile tea while practicing deep breathing for 5 minutes. Let the calming warmth settle into your body as you focus on the present moment.

Lavender (Lavandula angustifolia)

- Properties: Lavender is famous for its ability to calm the nervous system and bring the mind and body back into balance. Its grounding qualities help reduce anxiety and promote relaxation.
- How to Use: Use lavender essential oil in a diffuser to create a calming atmosphere in your home, or make a lavender sachet to place under your pillow for restful sleep.
- Practical Tip: Before bed, create a grounding ritual by rubbing a few drops of lavender essential oil on your temples and practicing a body scan meditation, focusing on each part of your body from head to toe.

Valerian (Valeriana officinalis)

- Properties: Valerian is a powerful herb for calming the nervous system and relieving restlessness or anxiety. It is often used to promote deep, restful sleep, making it ideal for grounding the mind and body at the end of the day.
- How to Use: Brew valerian root into a tea before bed to unwind, or take it as a supplement for a stronger effect.

- **Practical Tip:** Create a nightly grounding ritual by combining valerian tea with a few moments of reflection or journaling. Focus on letting go of the day's stresses as you prepare for sleep.

Grounding Rituals: Simple Practices for Everyday Life

Alongside these herbs, grounding rituals can help you reconnect with your body and center your mind. Here are a few simple practices you can incorporate into your daily life to feel more rooted and balanced:

Tea Meditation

- **How it Works:** Select one of the grounding teas (Chamomile, Lavender, or Valerian) and create a mindful tea-drinking ritual. As you brew the tea, focus on the scent, the warmth of the cup in your hands, and the flavor as you sip. Breathe deeply between sips, letting the experience calm and center you.
- **Why It's Effective:** This practice not only incorporates the grounding effects of the herbs but also invites you to be fully present in the moment, helping to reduce anxiety and stress.

Grounding Breath-Work

How it Works: Find a quiet space and sit comfortably with both feet planted on the ground. Take a few slow, deep breaths, inhaling for four counts and exhaling for six counts. As you breathe, imagine roots extending from the soles of your feet into the earth. Visualize these roots growing deeper with each breath, anchoring you to the ground beneath you.

Why It's Effective: This simple breath-work technique is a powerful way to ground yourself and create a sense of calm in moments of overwhelm.

Walking Barefoot in Nature

- How it Works: If possible, take off your shoes and walk barefoot on grass, soil, or sand. As you walk, focus on the sensation of the earth beneath your feet. Feel the connection between your body and the ground, letting the energy of the earth steady and center you.
- Why It's Effective: Walking barefoot, also known as "earthing," allows your body to connect directly with the earth's energy, helping to balance your nervous system and reduce stress.

Practical Tip: Creating a Grounding Ritual

Try incorporating a daily grounding ritual using a combination of these herbs and practices. Here's a simple routine to get started:

- Morning: Start your day with a grounding breath-work exercise to center yourself.
- Midday: Take a short break to walk outside, focusing on your connection to the earth.
- Evening: End your day with a cup of chamomile or valerian tea and a few minutes of mindful reflection or journaling.

Final Thoughts on Grounding:

Grounding is a practice that can be easily integrated into your daily life.

By incorporating these herbs and rituals, you'll find it easier to stay balanced, present, and calm, even during stressful times. Remember that healing starts with small, intentional steps, and grounding yourself is the foundation for all other forms of self-care.

2

Energizing Herbs for Body and Spirit

Why We Need Energy and Balance

We live in a world that asks so much of us—mentally, emotionally, and physically. Some days, just getting out of bed can feel like a monumental task. Whether it's work, family responsibilities, or the simple challenges of navigating daily life, it's easy to feel drained and depleted. But energy doesn't have to come from a cup of coffee or a quick fix. Nature provides us with gentle, sustainable ways to boost our vitality and bring our body and spirit back into balance.

In this section, we'll explore energizing herbs that not only restore your physical energy but also lift your mood and bring mental clarity. These herbs work with your body to naturally recharge, helping you move through your day with more lightness, focus, and ease.

Energizing Herbs: Uplifting and Restoring Vitality

Lemon (Citrus limon)

- Properties: Lemon is an energizing and revitalizing fruit that brings a burst of freshness to your body and mind. Its bright, citrus scent helps clear mental fog, uplift the mood, and refresh your spirit. Lemon also has detoxifying properties, making it great for recharging the body.
- How to Use: Add fresh lemon slices to water throughout the day for hydration and detoxification. You can also use lemon essential oil in a diffuser to brighten your home and lift your spirits.
- Practical Tip: Start your morning with a warm glass of lemon water. This simple ritual hydrates, detoxifies, and provides a gentle energy boost to help you start your day on the right foot.

Peppermint (Mentha piperita)

- Properties: Peppermint is known for its ability to invigorate and stimulate the mind. It boosts energy and alertness while also improving focus and concentration. The cooling sensation of peppermint can also help reduce physical fatigue and tension.
- How to Use: Brew peppermint tea for a refreshing midday energy boost, or apply diluted peppermint oil to your temples to relieve headaches and mental fatigue.
- Practical Tip: Try using peppermint tea as a facial steam to awaken your senses. Simply pour boiling water over a few peppermint leaves in a bowl, cover your head with a towel, and lean over the steam for a few minutes to clear your mind and refresh your spirit.

Rosemary (Rosmarinus officinalis)

- Properties: Rosemary is a powerful herb for enhancing memory, mental clarity, and concentration. It stimulates circulation and clears mental fog, making it perfect for times when you need focus and stamina.

- How to Use: Add fresh rosemary to your cooking, or brew rosemary tea for a refreshing, mind-clearing drink. You can also burn dried rosemary as an herbal incense to cleanse the air and enhance mental clarity.
- Practical Tip: Keep a small rosemary plant by your workspace. The scent alone can help keep your mind sharp and focused throughout the day.

Ginseng (Panax ginseng)

- Properties: Ginseng is a well-known adaptogen that helps the body adapt to stress while boosting energy and endurance. It's often used to combat fatigue and increase vitality, making it perfect for long-term energy support.
- How to Use: Ginseng is commonly taken as a tea or in capsule form. It's a great herb to add to your daily routine, especially when you need sustained energy throughout the day.
- Practical Tip: Start your day with a cup of ginseng tea for sustained energy, especially if you know you'll need to stay focused and alert for long periods of time.

Energizing Rituals: Simple Practices for Uplifting Your Energy

Incorporating herbs into your daily life is a great way to restore energy, but pairing them with energizing rituals takes it a step further. Here are some simple rituals that will help you recharge physically and mentally, using the power of both nature and intention.

Morning Citrus Ritual

- How it Works: Start your day with a warm glass of lemon water. Sit quietly for a few minutes as you sip, focusing on the sensations of warmth and citrus. Let the bright, fresh flavor awaken your senses and energize your body.
- Why It's Effective: This ritual not only hydrates and detoxifies your body, but the simple act of mindfulness in the morning helps you set a positive tone for the day ahead.

Peppermint Cooling Mist

- How it Works: Make a simple peppermint cooling mist by adding a few drops of peppermint essential oil to a spray bottle of water. Mist your face and neck throughout the day whenever you need a refreshing pick-me-up.
- Why It's Effective: Peppermint's cooling and invigorating properties will help reduce physical fatigue while also awakening your mind.

Lemon Balm Midday Reset

- How it Works: Brew a cup of lemon balm tea for a midday break. Sit outside or near a window, and take a few deep breaths as you sip, letting the gentle, uplifting properties of lemon balm calm your mind and refresh your energy.
- Why It's Effective: Lemon balm's stress-relieving properties help balance your mood and energy, providing mental clarity without overstimulation.

Rosemary Focus Meditation

- How it Works: Before starting a big project or task, take a few moments to inhale the scent of fresh rosemary or rosemary essential oil. Close your eyes, take three deep breaths, and imagine the herb clearing your mind, sharpening your focus, and giving you the mental stamina you need to complete your task.

- Why It's Effective: Rosemary's stimulating properties will help you stay focused and alert, while the meditation prepares your mind for clarity and concentration.

Practical Tip: Creating an Energizing Morning Routine

Begin each day with intention and vitality by combining energizing herbs and rituals. Here's a simple routine to help you feel refreshed and ready for the day:

- Morning Lemon Water: Start with a warm glass of lemon water to hydrate and awaken your senses.
- Peppermint Facial Steam: After your lemon water, treat yourself to a quick peppermint steam to clear your mind.
- Rosemary Focus Ritual: Before diving into work, inhale the scent of rosemary to sharpen your focus and set the tone for a productive, energized day.

Final Thoughts on Energy:

Energizing herbs and rituals are nature's way of helping us restore balance and vitality. By incorporating these practices into your daily routine, you can move through your day with more focus, ease, and energy—without the need for artificial stimulants. Remember, the key to sustainable energy is gentle, consistent nourishment, both for your body and your mind.

3

Herbal Support for Emotional Healing

Emotional Healing: Finding Balance in Times of Stress

Our emotions are powerful forces that shape how we experience the world, and when we are overwhelmed by stress, anxiety, or sadness, it can feel like we're caught in a storm with no anchor. While we all experience emotional ups and downs, finding tools to support our emotional wellness can make these difficult moments easier to navigate. Nature offers us healing herbs that gently calm the nervous system, soothe the heart, and bring us back to center.

In this section, we'll explore herbs that help release emotional tension, support mental wellness, and bring a sense of calm and balance during times of stress. These herbs work with the body and mind, helping to ease anxiety, lift your mood, and support emotional resilience.

Herbs for Emotional Healing: Calming and Soothing the Spirit

St. John's Wort (Hypericum perforatum)

- Properties: St. John's Wort is often used to help ease mild to moderate depression and uplift the mood. It works as a natural antidepressant by promoting serotonin production and helping to regulate emotions.
- How to Use: St. John's Wort can be taken as a tea or tincture. Consistent use over time helps to gradually lift the mood and reduce feelings of hopelessness or sadness.
- Practical Tip: Begin your day with a cup of St. John's Wort tea when you're feeling low or emotionally depleted. Use this as a moment of self-compassion, reminding yourself that healing is a process.

Ashwagandha (Withania somnifera)

- Properties: Ashwagandha is an adaptogen, which means it helps the body and mind adapt to stress. It's known for its ability to reduce anxiety, balance cortisol levels, and promote a sense of calm, making it ideal for emotional resilience.
- How to Use: Take ashwagandha in a capsule or tincture form daily to help balance your stress response over time. It can also be added to teas or smoothies.
- Practical Tip: Mix ashwagandha powder into a warm evening drink (like a spiced milk or tea) to create a soothing ritual before bed, helping you release the stress of the day.

Holy Basil (Ocimum sanctum)

- Properties: Also known as Tulsi, Holy Basil is a sacred herb that helps calm the mind and uplift the spirit. It's often used to reduce feelings of anxiety and emotional stress while promoting mental clarity and calmness.
- How to Use: Brew Holy Basil tea in the afternoon or evening when

you feel emotionally overwhelmed, or take it as a tincture during periods of intense stress.

- Practical Tip: Create a simple Holy Basil tea ceremony, taking a few minutes to sip slowly and reflect on what emotions are weighing you down. Breathe deeply and let the tea guide you back to a place of calm.

Lemon Balm (Melissa officinalis)

- Properties: Lemon Balm is a gentle yet powerful herb that supports emotional healing by calming the nervous system and reducing feelings of stress and anxiety. Its light, uplifting scent and flavor also help boost the mood.
- How to Use: Lemon Balm is best enjoyed as a tea, tincture, or aromatherapy oil. Its calming properties make it an ideal herb to incorporate into your daily routine, especially during moments of emotional tension.
- Practical Tip: Use lemon balm in a self-care ritual—prepare a cup of lemon balm tea and pair it with deep breathing exercises to release built-up emotional tension.

Passionflower (Passiflora incarnata)

- Properties: Passionflower is known for its calming effects, making it an excellent herb for reducing anxiety and quieting an overactive mind. It gently helps relax the body and promotes restful sleep, especially for those who struggle with racing thoughts or stress-induced insomnia.
- How to Use: Brew passionflower into a tea for deep relaxation before bed, or take it as a tincture during stressful periods to calm the mind.
- Practical Tip: At the end of a stressful day, steep a cup of passion-

flower tea and allow yourself to unwind. Pair it with a gratitude journaling exercise to shift your focus from stress to the things in your life that bring you peace and joy.

Emotional Healing Rituals: Nurturing the Mind and Spirit

Incorporating emotional healing rituals into your life helps to process feelings, reduce stress, and bring a sense of balance and emotional resilience. Here are a few gentle practices to support emotional well-being using herbs and simple rituals.

Evening Reflection and Tea Ritual

- How it Works: Choose a calming herb, such as lemon balm or passionflower, and brew a cup of tea in the evening. As you sip, take a few moments to reflect on the emotions of the day. What emotions came up? What are you ready to release? Allow the herb's calming properties to guide you as you reflect and release emotional tension.
- Why It's Effective: This simple practice helps you unwind at the end of the day, giving you space to process emotions while using calming herbs to bring your nervous system back into balance.

Herbal Bath for Emotional Release

- How it Works: Create an herbal bath by adding dried lavender, chamomile, and a few drops of lavender essential oil to warm bath water. As you soak, imagine the water washing away emotional stress and tension. Focus on your breathing and let yourself feel nurtured by the warmth and healing properties of the herbs.

- Why It's Effective: Water is a powerful tool for emotional cleansing, and when combined with herbs, it becomes a sacred space for letting go of heavy emotions.

Holy Basil Morning Meditation

- How it Works: Start your morning with a cup of Holy Basil tea, and as you sip, practice a short, gentle meditation. Close your eyes, focus on your breath, and set an emotional intention for the day. Perhaps you choose peace, clarity, or patience. Let the herb support you in maintaining this emotional state throughout the day.
- Why It's Effective: Setting an emotional intention each morning helps you move through the day with purpose, and Holy Basil's calming properties support emotional resilience as you encounter challenges.

Ashwagandha Stress-Relief Ritual

- How it Works: Prepare a warm, soothing drink with ashwagandha powder (such as golden milk or spiced tea) before bed. Sit quietly in a comfortable space and take a few slow, deep breaths, focusing on releasing the stress of the day. Allow the adaptogenic properties of ashwagandha to support your body's stress response as you wind down.
- Why It's Effective: This ritual helps your body let go of physical and emotional stress, allowing you to sleep more peacefully and reset for the day ahead.

Practical Tip: Creating an Emotional Healing Routine

Emotional healing requires regular practice, just like physical healing. Start by creating a weekly emotional check-in routine:

- Evening Tea Ritual: Dedicate one evening per week to brewing a calming tea, reflecting on your emotions, and journaling what you're ready to release.
- Midweek Stress Reset: Incorporate a short meditation or breathing exercise with Holy Basil tea or passionflower tincture midweek to restore emotional balance.
- Herbal Bath Ritual: Once a month, treat yourself to an herbal bath to cleanse your body and mind of emotional stress.

Final Thoughts on Emotional Healing:

Emotional healing is a lifelong journey, but it doesn't have to be overwhelming. By using herbs that calm the mind and soothe the heart, combined with simple, intentional rituals, you can navigate difficult emotions with more ease and grace. Let these practices be your anchor when life feels heavy, and remember that healing is a process that takes time, patience, and self-compassion.

4

Immune-Boosting Herbs and Rituals

Supporting the Immune System Naturally

Our immune system works tirelessly to protect us from illness and keep our bodies functioning at their best. But just like any part of our body, it needs regular care and nourishment. When we feel run down, stressed, or overwhelmed, our immune system can become compromised, leaving us vulnerable to sickness. Fortunately, nature provides us with powerful herbs that help support our immunity, allowing us to stay strong and resilient throughout the year.

In this section, we'll explore herbs that strengthen the immune system, support the body during seasonal changes, and help you recover more quickly from illness. Paired with simple self-care rituals, these immune-boosting practices will help you feel grounded, nourished, and ready to take on whatever life brings.

Herbs for Immune Support: Strengthening the Body's Defenses

Elderberry (Sambucus nigra)

- Properties: Elderberry is one of the most well-known herbs for boosting the immune system. Rich in antioxidants and vitamin C, elderberry helps to strengthen the body's natural defenses and is especially helpful during cold and flu season.
- How to Use: Elderberry is commonly made into syrups, teas, and tinctures. You can take it daily as a preventative measure or use it at the onset of illness to shorten recovery time.
- Practical Tip: Make a simple elderberry syrup to take daily during the winter months. Combine elderberries, honey, and water in a pot, simmer, strain, and store in the fridge. Take a spoonful each morning to help strengthen your immune system.

Echinacea (Echinacea purpurea)

- Properties: Echinacea is a powerful herb that stimulates the immune system, helping the body fight off infections. It's particularly effective when taken at the first sign of illness, as it can reduce the severity and duration of colds and flu.
- How to Use: Echinacea is available in teas, tinctures, and capsules. For best results, use it at the first sign of illness to help your body ward off infection.
- Practical Tip: Brew a cup of echinacea tea when you feel a cold coming on. Pair it with a few moments of rest, allowing your body to focus on healing.

Ginger (Zingiber officinale)

- Properties: Ginger is not only a powerful anti-inflammatory but also a warming herb that helps the body fight off infections and soothe respiratory issues. It's commonly used for colds, flu, and digestive support, making it a great all-around immune booster.

- How to Use: Ginger can be brewed into tea, added to soups and broths, or taken in capsule form. Fresh ginger tea is especially effective for soothing a sore throat or clearing congestion.
- Practical Tip: Start your day with a warm cup of fresh ginger tea. Boil sliced ginger root in water for 10 minutes, strain, and add a squeeze of lemon and honey for an added immune boost.

Turmeric (Curcuma longa)

- Properties: Turmeric is a potent anti-inflammatory and antioxidant-rich herb that supports the immune system and overall wellness. It helps reduce inflammation in the body and protects against chronic illness, making it an essential herb for long-term immune health.
- How to Use: Turmeric is commonly used in teas, golden milk, or as a spice in cooking. You can also take it as a supplement for concentrated immune support.
- Practical Tip: Try making a soothing turmeric latte, also known as golden milk. Combine turmeric powder with warm milk (or a plant-based alternative), a pinch of black pepper, and honey for a comforting immune-boosting drink before bed.

Astragalus (Astragalus membranaceus)

- Properties: Astragalus is an adaptogen that helps strengthen the immune system and increase the body's resistance to stress and illness. It's especially effective for preventing illness during times of seasonal change or when you're feeling run down.
- How to Use: Astragalus is typically taken as a tea or tincture. It can also be added to soups and broths for a nourishing, immune-boosting meal.
- Practical Tip: Add a few slices of dried astragalus root to your next

batch of vegetable or bone broth. Let it simmer to extract its immune-boosting properties, then strain and enjoy a cup when you're feeling under the weather.

Immune-Boosting Rituals: Caring for Your Body During Seasonal Changes

Herbs are powerful allies for your immune system, but pairing them with self-care rituals can take your immunity to the next level. These immune-boosting rituals help you stay resilient during times of stress or seasonal changes, giving your body the support it needs to stay strong and healthy.

Daily Herbal Tonic for Immune Support

- How it Works: Prepare a daily immune-boosting tonic using elderberry syrup, ginger, and lemon. Mix a spoonful of elderberry syrup with warm water, a slice of fresh ginger, and a squeeze of lemon. Sip this tonic in the morning to support your immune system throughout the day.
- Why It's Effective: This combination of herbs provides antioxidants, anti-inflammatory properties, and vitamin C, giving your immune system the tools it needs to stay strong.

Herbal Steam for Congestion Relief

- How it Works: When you're feeling congested or under the weather, prepare an herbal steam using fresh ginger and eucalyptus oil. Boil water with slices of ginger, pour into a bowl, and add a few drops of eucalyptus oil. Place a towel over your head and breathe deeply over the steam for 5–10 minutes.

- Why It's Effective: This ritual helps clear your sinuses, soothes respiratory issues, and boosts circulation, making it easier for your body to fight off infections.

Turmeric and Ginger Warming Tea

- How it Works: Create a warming tea using fresh ginger and turmeric to soothe inflammation and support your immune system. Boil water with slices of ginger and turmeric root, strain, and add honey to taste. Drink this tea when you're feeling run down or during cold and flu season.
- Why It's Effective: Ginger and turmeric are both powerful anti-inflammatory herbs that help reduce swelling, support digestion, and fight off infections, making them ideal for immune health.

Restorative Herbal Bath

- How it Works: Draw a warm bath and add a handful of Epsom salts, dried lavender, and a few drops of eucalyptus essential oil. As you soak, focus on your breath and allow the warm water and herbs to soothe your body and release tension.
- Why It's Effective: This ritual not only helps reduce physical tension but also supports your immune system by helping your body relax and reset.

Practical Tip: Creating an Immune-Boosting Routine

During cold and flu season or times of increased stress, it's important to give your immune system extra support. Here's a simple immune-boosting routine you can follow:

- Morning: Start your day with a daily herbal tonic, mixing elderberry syrup with warm water, lemon, and ginger.
- Midday: Take a break for a cup of turmeric and ginger tea, allowing the anti-inflammatory properties to nourish your body.
- Evening: Draw a warm, restorative herbal bath with Epsom salts, eucalyptus oil, and lavender to help your body unwind and recover.

Final Thoughts on Immune Health:

Supporting your immune system is about more than just avoiding illness—it's about giving your body the tools it needs to stay balanced, strong, and resilient. By incorporating these immune-boosting herbs and simple rituals into your daily life, you can protect your health, recover more quickly from illness, and maintain overall wellness no matter the season.

5

Herbs for Sleep and Rest

The Importance of Rest and Sleep

Sleep is one of the most vital components of overall health, yet it's often the first thing to suffer when life gets busy or stressful. Without adequate rest, our bodies and minds struggle to function at their best. Poor sleep can lead to heightened stress, decreased immune function, and emotional imbalances. The good news is that nature provides a range of herbs that gently encourage relaxation, calm the mind, and promote restful, restorative sleep.

In this section, we'll explore herbs that soothe the nervous system, reduce anxiety, and help you drift into a deep, peaceful sleep. Paired with calming evening rituals, these herbs will help you establish a healthy bedtime routine, allowing you to wake up feeling refreshed and restored.

Herbs for Sleep: Calming and Restorative

Passionflower (Passiflora incarnata)

- Properties: Passionflower is a powerful herb for calming an overactive mind, making it perfect for those who have trouble falling asleep due to racing thoughts or anxiety. It relaxes the nervous system and helps ease the transition into sleep.
- How to Use: Brew passionflower into a tea before bed, or take it as a tincture for stronger effects. It's especially helpful for those who experience stress-induced insomnia.
- Practical Tip: Make a habit of enjoying a cup of passionflower tea in the evening, paired with a relaxation exercise such as gentle stretching or breathing, to help quiet your mind before bed.

Chamomile (Matricaria chamomilla)

- Properties: Chamomile is well known for its soothing and calming effects. It gently relaxes the muscles and the mind, making it an ideal herb for promoting restful sleep and reducing nighttime anxiety.
- How to Use: Chamomile tea is a classic nighttime remedy. Sip a warm cup of tea before bed to relax your body and prepare for sleep.
- Practical Tip: Brew a cup of chamomile tea and sip it while reading or journaling before bed. Use this time to unwind and reflect, allowing chamomile to help your body shift into relaxation mode.

Valerian (Valeriana officinalis)

- Properties: Valerian is a strong herbal sedative, commonly used to treat insomnia and restlessness. It calms the nervous system and promotes deep, restorative sleep, especially for those who have trouble staying asleep through the night.
- How to Use: Take valerian as a tincture or capsule 30 minutes before bed. Due to its strong taste, many people prefer tinctures or capsules over tea.

- Practical Tip: If you struggle with insomnia, try taking valerian in the evening and pairing it with a calming bath to further relax your body and mind before sleep.

Lemon Balm (Melissa officinalis)

- Properties: Lemon balm is a gentle herb that calms the nervous system and reduces anxiety. Its mild sedative effects help the mind wind down, making it a perfect herb for promoting restful sleep, especially when combined with other calming herbs.
- How to Use: Lemon balm can be taken as a tea or tincture in the evening. It pairs well with chamomile and passionflower for a soothing nighttime blend.
- Practical Tip: Create a calming nighttime tea blend by combining lemon balm with chamomile and passionflower. Enjoy this tea about an hour before bed to give your body time to relax and prepare for sleep.

Lavender (Lavandula angustifolia)

- Properties: Lavender is widely known for its calming aroma, which helps reduce anxiety and promotes relaxation. It is commonly used to support sleep by soothing the nervous system and easing stress.
- How to Use: Use lavender essential oil in a diffuser in your bedroom, or make a lavender sachet to place under your pillow for restful sleep.
- Practical Tip: Add a few drops of lavender essential oil to your pillow before bed. Inhale deeply as you lie down, focusing on the soothing scent and allowing it to calm your mind and body.

Sleep and Rest Rituals: Preparing the Body and Mind for Deep Sleep

Incorporating calming herbs into your evening routine is a wonderful way to promote restful sleep, but pairing them with soothing rituals can enhance their effects. These simple bedtime rituals will help you wind down from the day, reduce stress, and prepare for deep, restorative sleep.

Herbal Sleep Tea and Journal Reflection

- How it Works: About an hour before bed, brew a cup of calming herbal tea (such as a blend of chamomile, lemon balm, and passionflower). As you sip, spend a few minutes reflecting on your day in a journal. Write down anything that's on your mind—what went well, what's worrying you—so that you can clear your head before sleep.
- Why It's Effective: This combination of herbal tea and journaling helps calm both the body and mind. Writing down your thoughts allows you to release any mental tension, while the herbs relax your nervous system, preparing you for a peaceful night's sleep.

Lavender Sleep Mist

- How it Works: Make a simple lavender sleep mist by combining water and a few drops of lavender essential oil in a spray bottle. Spritz your pillow, bed linens, and bedroom before bedtime to create a calming, restful atmosphere.
- Why It's Effective: Lavender's soothing aroma helps signal to your brain that it's time to relax and wind down. This ritual helps create a tranquil sleep environment, encouraging your mind and body to let go of the day's stress.

Evening Bath for Deep Relaxation

- How it Works: About an hour before bed, draw a warm bath and add Epsom salts and a few drops of lavender or chamomile essential oil. As you soak, focus on your breathing, allowing your body to relax fully. Let the warmth of the water and the soothing aroma of the herbs ease away tension and prepare your body for sleep.
- Why It's Effective: A warm bath not only relaxes your muscles but also helps signal to your nervous system that it's time to rest. The addition of calming herbs helps enhance this relaxation, making it easier to fall asleep and stay asleep.

Valerian Restful Sleep Ritual

- How it Works: If you struggle with insomnia, try taking valerian tincture or capsules about 30 minutes before bed. Pair this with a brief meditation or breathing exercise, focusing on relaxing your body from head to toe. As you breathe deeply, visualize your body releasing the day's stress and tension.
- Why It's Effective: Valerian is a strong sedative herb, and when paired with relaxation techniques, it helps the body and mind fully prepare for sleep. This ritual is particularly helpful for those who find it difficult to fall or stay asleep.

Practical Tip: Creating a Calming Bedtime Routine

A consistent bedtime routine is essential for promoting restful sleep. Here's a simple nighttime routine to help you wind down and prepare for deep, restorative sleep:

- Evening Tea: About an hour before bed, brew a cup of chamomile or

passionflower tea to start relaxing your body and mind.
- Lavender Sleep Mist: Spray your pillow and linens with lavender sleep mist to create a calming atmosphere.
- Bath or Meditation: Take a warm bath or spend a few minutes in quiet meditation, focusing on releasing the day's stress and preparing your body for rest.

Final Thoughts on Sleep and Rest:

A good night's sleep is one of the greatest gifts you can give yourself. By incorporating these calming herbs and simple bedtime rituals into your evening routine, you can create a peaceful space for your body and mind to rest and recharge. Sleep is the foundation for emotional and physical well-being, and with the support of nature's gentle remedies, you can enjoy deeper, more restorative sleep each night.

6

Skin and Body Wellness with Herbs

Nurturing Your Skin and Body Naturally

Our skin is not only our body's largest organ but also a mirror reflecting our overall health and well-being. Just as we nourish our bodies from the inside, the skin also benefits from natural, holistic care that comes directly from nature. Using herbs to nurture the skin not only addresses surface concerns but also promotes deeper healing by working with the body's natural processes.

In this section, we'll explore herbs that support healthy, radiant skin, promote healing, and soothe irritation. These herbs, paired with simple self-care rituals, will help you create nourishing routines that leave your skin feeling rejuvenated, hydrated, and balanced.

Herbs for Skin and Body Wellness: Nourishing, Healing, and Protecting

Calendula (Calendula officinalis)

- Properties: Calendula is a soothing and healing herb often used to treat dry, irritated, or damaged skin. Its anti-inflammatory and antimicrobial properties help speed up healing, making it ideal for cuts, scrapes, and skin conditions like eczema.
- How to Use: Infuse calendula flowers in oil to create a healing balm or use calendula-infused oil directly on the skin for nourishment and repair.
- Practical Tip: Make a simple calendula salve by infusing dried calendula flowers in olive oil, then blending with beeswax for a soothing, all-purpose skin balm.

Aloe Vera (Aloe barbadensis)

- Properties: Aloe vera is well known for its cooling and soothing properties, making it perfect for sunburns, rashes, and irritated skin. It hydrates and heals the skin while reducing redness and inflammation.
- How to Use: Apply fresh aloe vera gel directly to the skin or use aloe-infused products for a quick, cooling treatment.
- Practical Tip: Keep a small aloe vera plant at home. Break off a leaf to extract the fresh gel whenever you need to soothe a sunburn, rash, or irritation.

Rose (Rosa damascena)

- Properties: Rose is a deeply nourishing and hydrating herb that helps soothe and balance the skin. It's known for its anti-inflammatory properties and ability to reduce redness, making it ideal for sensitive or mature skin.
- How to Use: Rose can be used in skincare as a hydrosol (rosewater), in oils, or as an infused bath herb. Rose-infused oil can be used to

moisturize and protect the skin.

- Practical Tip: Make a refreshing rosewater mist by combining rose hydrosol with a few drops of rose essential oil in a spray bottle. Mist your face throughout the day for a gentle, hydrating boost.

Lavender (Lavandula angustifolia)

- Properties: Lavender is a versatile herb that soothes irritated skin, reduces inflammation, and promotes healing. It's often used to treat acne, rashes, and minor burns while also calming the mind and body.
- How to Use: Use lavender essential oil in homemade skincare products, or add dried lavender to a relaxing bath to soothe both skin and mind.
- Practical Tip: Add a few drops of lavender essential oil to your favorite moisturizer or body lotion to enhance its calming and healing properties, especially if your skin is feeling stressed or irritated.

Comfrey (Symphytum officinale)

- Properties: Comfrey is known for its powerful skin-healing abilities. It contains allantoin, a compound that promotes cell regeneration and speeds up the healing of wounds, making it great for scrapes, burns, and other skin irritations.
- How to Use: Create a comfrey-infused oil or balm to apply to cuts, scrapes, and irritated skin. It can also be used as a poultice for deeper healing.
- Practical Tip: Use comfrey-infused oil as a part of your daily skincare routine, especially for dry or damaged skin. Apply to areas that need extra healing, such as rough patches or scars.

Body Wellness Rituals: Caring for Your Skin and Body Naturally

Herbs can provide deep nourishment for the skin and body, but pairing them with self-care rituals enhances their healing benefits. These simple, holistic rituals help you connect with your body and nourish your skin in a gentle, intentional way.

Herbal Face Steam for Glowing Skin

- How it Works: Create a simple herbal face steam using dried lavender, chamomile, and rose petals. Boil water, pour it into a bowl, and add the herbs. Drape a towel over your head and lean over the steam, allowing it to open your pores and refresh your skin.
- Why It's Effective: Herbal steams help cleanse the pores and allow the skin to absorb the beneficial properties of the herbs. This ritual also promotes relaxation, making it an excellent way to care for both your skin and your mental well-being.

Nourishing Herbal Body Scrub

- How it Works: Make a gentle body scrub using sugar, coconut oil, and dried herbs such as calendula and lavender. Massage the scrub into your skin in circular motions, focusing on areas that need extra exfoliation.
- Why It's Effective: Exfoliating the skin helps remove dead skin cells and promotes circulation, while the herbs nourish and soothe the skin. This ritual leaves your skin feeling smooth, refreshed, and deeply moisturized.

Soothing Herbal Bath Soak

- How it Works: Prepare a warm bath with a handful of dried calendula, rose petals, and lavender, along with a few tablespoons of Epsom salts. Soak for at least 20 minutes, allowing the herbs to calm your skin and mind.
- Why It's Effective: Herbal baths are a wonderful way to nourish the skin while relaxing the body. The combination of herbs and warm water soothes irritation, promotes healing, and helps reduce stress.

DIY Herbal Body Oil

- How it Works: Infuse olive oil or jojoba oil with dried calendula, rose petals, or lavender for 4-6 weeks, then strain and use as a daily body oil. After a shower, massage the oil into your skin to lock in moisture and nourish your body.
- Why It's Effective: Herbal-infused oils are rich in nutrients and antioxidants that deeply nourish the skin, leaving it hydrated, smooth, and protected. Regular use helps improve skin texture and overall health.

Practical Tip: Creating a Weekly Skin and Body Wellness Routine

To keep your skin healthy and glowing, incorporate a simple, natural skincare routine into your week:

- Midweek Face Steam: Give your skin a refresh with a midweek herbal face steam, using lavender and chamomile to open your pores and soothe irritation.
- Weekend Body Scrub: Treat yourself to a nourishing body scrub on the weekend, exfoliating and moisturizing your skin to keep it

smooth and radiant.

- Herbal Body Oil: After every shower, massage a herbal-infused body oil into your skin to lock in moisture and nourish your body.

Final Thoughts on Skin and Body Wellness:

Taking care of your skin is about more than just beauty—it's about nourishing your body from the outside in, using the gentle power of herbs to support health and wellness. By incorporating these herbs and simple rituals into your routine, you can cultivate healthy, radiant skin that reflects your overall well-being. Remember, caring for your body is an act of self-love, and with nature's help, you can nourish yourself every day.

7

Conclusion

Embracing Your Healing Journey

As you've explored these pages, you've been introduced to the gentle wisdom of herbs and the transformative power of rituals. My hope is that these simple practices become a part of your daily life, guiding you toward deeper connection, healing, and balance.

Healing is not about perfection—it's about honoring where you are and giving yourself permission to grow and evolve, one step at a time. The herbs and rituals in this guide are tools to help you on that journey. They offer nourishment not only for the body but for the mind and spirit as well. Whether you're grounding yourself with calming herbs, boosting your energy naturally, or nurturing your skin, these practices remind you that nature is always there, ready to support you.

Remember, healing doesn't happen overnight, and it doesn't follow a straight line. It's a process of becoming—of learning to trust your body, care for your mind, and love yourself through every stage of the journey. The path to wellness is as unique as you are, and there's no rush to reach the finish line.

As you continue your journey, take time to reflect on what brings you peace, what makes you feel connected, and what helps you stay grounded. Healing is a lifelong practice, and you have everything you need to walk this path with grace, strength, and love.

Moving Forward with Nature's Support

As you carry these herbal remedies and rituals into your life, remember that the small, intentional steps you take today create a foundation for long-lasting wellness. Whether it's a daily cup of tea, a grounding meditation, or a calming bath at the end of a long day, these simple acts of care are powerful.

And, just as nature is always evolving and adapting, so too will your healing journey. Be patient with yourself, trust in the process, and know that every small step is a step toward wholeness.

Thank you for allowing me to share this guide with you. May the wisdom of nature, the support of these herbs, and the power of your own self-care carry you forward on your path of healing.

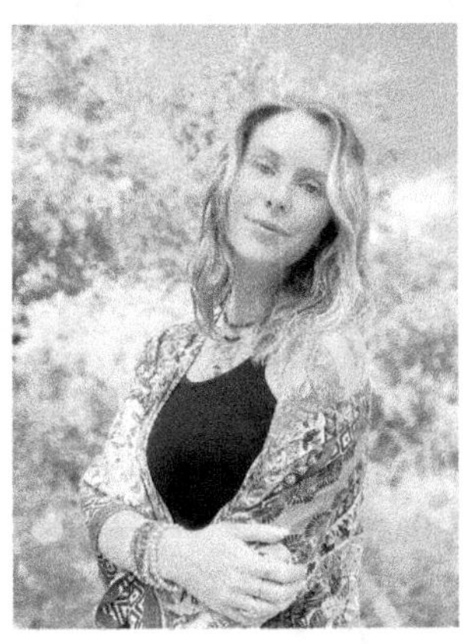

About the Author

Samantha Peterein is the founder of Luna & Daisy Herbal Co. LLC, a woman-owned small business rooted in nature and community. A lover of plants and holistic wellness, Samantha has dedicated her journey to healing—both personal and collective. Through her own experiences with loss, anxiety, and illness, she discovered the profound power of herbs and self-care rituals to restore balance and well-being.

Combining her deep connection to the earth with a passion for nurturing others, Samantha shares the wisdom of natural healing through her products and teachings. Her mission is to help individuals reconnect with themselves, embrace self-care, and find healing in everyday rituals.

When she's not working with herbs, you can find Samantha spending time in nature, creating new wellness products, and guiding her community toward a more balanced, holistic life.